Prostate Cancer
and the
Veteran

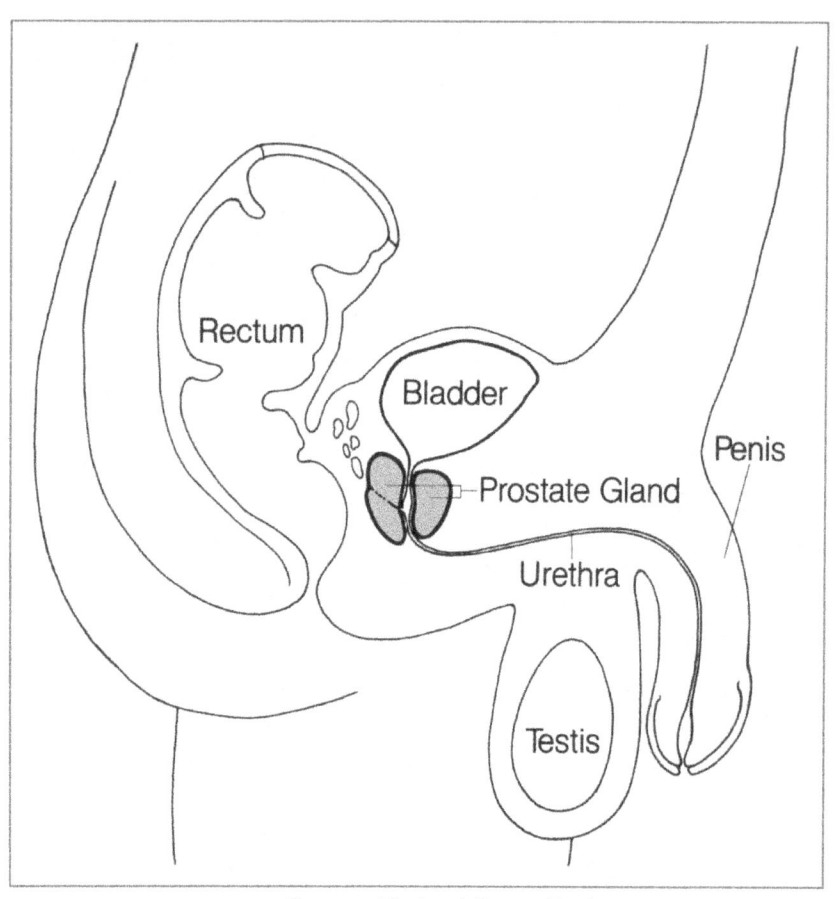

Courtesy National Cancer Institute

PROSTATE CANCER AND THE VETERAN

by

Tom Benjey

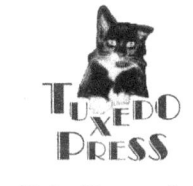

Carlisle, Pennsylvania

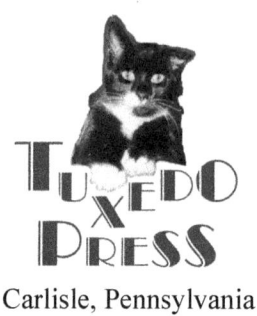

Carlisle, Pennsylvania

Copyright © 2011 by Tom Benjey

Published by Tuxedo Press
Carlisle, PA 17015
www.Tuxedo-Press.com

Cover photograph © David L. Terry

All rights reserved. No part of this publication may be reproduced, stored in a retrieval system, or transmitted, in any form or by any means, electronic, mechanical, photocopying, recording, or otherwise, without the prior permission of Tuxedo Press.

ISBN 978-1-936161-03-4

Table of Contents

Introduction 1
1 What You Need to Do Today 3
   I. You have been diagnosed with Prostate Cancer 3
   II. You Have Not Been Diagnosed with Prostate Cancer .. 6
2 My Story 9
3 VA Disabilities 21
   I. Agent Orange Diseases 21
   II. Disability Payments 24
4 Treatment Modalities for Prostate Cancer 29
   I. Watchful Waiting 30
   II. Surgery (Radical Prostatectomy) 30
   III. External Beam Radiation 31
   IV. Brachytherapy 32
   V. Cryotherapy 32
   VI. Proton Therapy 33
5 Cost 35
6 Conclusions 39

Introduction

The purpose of this guide is to share what I have learned about dealing with Prostate Cancer with other veterans, with an emphasis on Vietnam vets because of the Agent Orange issue. Not being a professional in any of the areas other than that of being a patient, my advice is based on personal experience and cannot be substituted for that of trained professionals. However, it might be useful in helping you formulate questions to ask the professionals. The government provides disability benefits to veterans whose Prostate Cancer has been determined to have been a result of their military service. Proving that may be a relatively simple matter for those who served on the ground in Vietnam during the period Agent Orange was being used. It's almost as simple for some others who served in particular places at particular times as outlined later in this document. But for many, proving that your cancer is service-connected may be difficult, if not impossible. In any case, the government doesn't inform veterans that they are eligible for disability benefits for Prostate Cancer; they must find that out for themselves. This guide informs veterans with, or who might get, Prostate Cancer about the existence of VA disability payments that they may be entitled to for their service to the country.

After jump-starting those who have already been diagnosed with Prostate Cancer to take immediate action, the guide begins with a telling of the author's own experiences, not because they are unusual but because they are likely to be relatively similar to many others' experiences with some variance in the details. It then provides information on the VA Disability benefits that are available as of this writing. Annual increases have been kept at 2009 levels in 2011 but may increase in the future. The third section discusses the various treatment modalities that are available for Prostate Cancer, along with their advantages and disadvantages. Choosing a course of treatment is a very personal decision. The aim of this guide is to provide an overview of these treatments so that you know they exist and can explore the ones that seem most suitable for your situation. The final section is a discussion of the cost of the treatment, health insurance issues, and tax deductions. The material in this guide is dated as of the writing, but it is the author's intent to update it periodically as significant changes take place.

If you are a Vietnam veteran who has already been diagnosed with Prostate Cancer, you need to take action today. Start by reading the next section titled "What You Need to Do Today" and do the things specified in that section TODAY! When you finish that, you can read the rest of this guide. Others can skip to the section that follows it, at least for now.

If you find dealing with the Internet or filling out the forms to be daunting tasks, there is help in human form available to you. Many counties now have veterans service offices that can help you deal with the VA. If you live far from one of these offices, veteran service organizations that can also help may be closer to you. Follows is contact information for several organizations that can assist in dealing with the VA. In addition, there are a number of other, lesser-known, veteran organizations that can be of help.

- American Legion: 1-800-433-3318 or www.legion.org
- AMVETS: 1-877-726-8387
- Armed Forces Services Corporation: 1-888-237-2872 or www.afsc-usa.com
- Disabled American Veterans: 1-877-426-2838 or www.doc.org
- Paralyzed Veterans of America: 1-800-424-8200 or www.pva.org
- Veterans of Foreign Wars: 1-800-VFW-1988 or www.vfw.org
- Viet Nam Veterans of America: 1-800-882-1316 or www.vva.org

African-Americans, veterans and otherwise, may find this book helpful because of the higher incidence of prostate cancer in this group than the general population.

1
What You Need to Do Today

The following are steps you should take today if you, the veteran, have been diagnosed with Prostate Cancer. If you haven't been diagnosed, jump to II to see what you should do right now.

I. You have been diagnosed with Prostate Cancer

A. Request copies of all diagnoses, lab tests and other pertinent documents from your physician and urologist. These documents are needed to show that you have indeed been diagnosed with Prostate Cancer. The VA needs to know for sure that you have the disease before they will compensate you for it.

B. Request copies of the records in your military file from the appropriate agency. If you didn't keep copies yourself, this is a way of gathering up what is hopefully the bulk of them. Military records for all branches are kept at:

> National Personnel Records Center
> Military Personnel Records
> 9700 Page Avenue
> St. Louis, MO 63132-5100

Veterans or the next of kin of deceased veterans can request copies of their files on-line at vetrecs.archives.gov. All others must submit completed and signed copies of Standard Form 180 through the mail only. If you don't have your DD-214, it can be obtained separately and more quickly from the rest of your records. It can also be requested through vetrecs.archives.gov.

Some important records, such as orders that sent you to Vietnam, may be missing. You may need to be creative in figuring out ways to find copies of what you need. In my case, I wracked my brain until I remembered the name of a Tech Sergeant from my shop who traveled with me to Bien Hoa Air Base. All I had to do then was figure out how to spell his name correctly and find him using zabasearch.com. You might have to do something similar. The VA apparently accepts "buddy statements," letters from guys with whom you served who attest that you were there. It helps if they have records that prove they were where they say you were. Don't sit around waiting for the records to file your claim; file your claim today, even if you don't have everything in hand to support it because the date you file, even if incomplete, determines when benefits ultimately begin.

C. File for Disability Compensation from the Veterans Administration. The words "Disability Compensation" are important. The VA has numerous programs, some with names that sound like they would be applicable to you, but this is the correct one. You have three ways to apply: on-line immediately; print paper forms from a VA website, complete them and mail in them to the VA; or get forms from your local veterans service office, fill them out and mail them in to the VA. Let's start with the on-line application.

On the VA's website, www.va.gov, select VONAPP (Veterans On-line Application). VONAPP allows you to file your claim on-line without going through the hassle of printing legibly or typing on paper forms. It also helps get your application into the VA system quicker. The date your application is filed often establishes the start date for compensation for a disability.

VONAPP allows you to attach up to five files to it. Of course, the paper forms have to be scanned into digital format before attaching them. I suggest scanning them into PDF format because PDFs are widely used and can be printed or enlarged on the screen for easy viewing. I also suggest scanning each form into a separate file to eliminate confusion. All the pages of a multi-page form should be scanned into a single file in page order. I also suggest naming the files with your name and the form number. For example, my DD-214 file would be named Benjey, Thomas R. DD-214.PDF.

If you are not comfortable printing out forms from Internet websites, ask your local veterans service office for assistance in filing your claim. Such groups can also help with problems in dealing with the VA. To print out the application form, go to www.va.gov and click on the VA Forms button (on the right side of the screen as of this writing). A form selection window will appear on which there is a Form Number box. Key in 21-526 to cause the desired PDF to display. Print the entire form including the instruction pages on your printer. Follow the instructions closely when filling out the form. Most veterans with Prostate Cancer will be applying for Compensation Benefits. When finished, mail it to the closest VA Regional Office. Again, feel free to get advice from your local veterans service office whichever route you choose to apply.

D. When you file your claim, include all the ailments that you think are service-connected. They may not come into play at first because I have read that the VA initially assigns veterans with Prostate Cancer a 100% disability, the maximum possible regardless of how many things are wrong with you. Six months after treatment is completed, the VA will re-examine you to determine your level of disability at that time. If the cancer is gone, the level of disability is determined by residual damage of the disease or its treatment. Incontinence, impotence, frequent urination and waking to urinate occur commonly in "cured" patients and are awarded disability percentages depending on their severity. It is at this point that disabilities unrelated to Prostate Cancer can come into play, assuming that the Prostate Cancer has not left you 100% disabled.

E. Start educating yourself about Prostate Cancer and the various treatment modalities so that you can make an informed decision when you select a treatment.

Now that you have filed your claim with the VA, you can take the time to get a better handle on what is going on and what you must do. As a bonus, you can skip the next section.

II. You Have Not Been Diagnosed with Prostate Cancer

A. Get a PSA Test taken today! That way your physicians will have a baseline against which to compare with tests in later years. Veterans as young as 40 should get a baseline test because veterans are more likely to have Prostate Cancer than are other American males. And Vietnam veterans aren't the only ones at risk.

B. Request copies of the records in your military file from the appropriate agency. If you didn't keep copies yourself, this is a way of determining which ones the government can't easily lay their hands on. If they're missing important ones, it will give you time to find copies of the important ones before you need them. Military records for all branches are kept at:

> National Personnel Records Center
> Military Personnel Records
> 9700 Page Avenue
> St. Louis, MO 63132-5100

> Veterans or the next of kin of deceased veterans can request copies of their files on-line at vetrecs.archives.gov. All others must submit completed and signed copies of Standard Form 180 through the mail only. If you don't have your DD-214, it can be obtained separately from the rest of your records and more quickly. It can also be requested through vetrecs.archives.gov.

C. Review your medical records to determine if any health conditions you currently have are service connected. Chances are that you have some relatively minor service-connected injury or disease that does not qualify you for more than a tiny disability rating, if any at all, but getting it on the books could be beneficial later. In my case, Tinnitus had been documented in my records as far back as 1968. By itself, it is something like a 10% disability and compensations are not computed proportionally. That is, a 10% disability is not compensated at 10% of the amount of a 100% disability. According to the VA's 2010 table (which is currently in use in 2011), a 100% disability is compensated at $2,673 a month but a veteran with a 10% disability is only paid $123 per month, 4.6% of the full amount. In addition, veterans with disabilities of 30% or more are eligible to receive additional compensation if they are married, have dependent children, or have dependent parents. The VA has tables which spell out the various amounts for each disability percentage with and without dependents. These dollar amounts can vary year by year but have been stable recently.

Even small dollar amounts can add up over the years; multiple small disabilities can be added together to create larger percentages. As our bodies decay over time, problems can surface that create disabilities that we didn't have when we were younger. A few relatively small disabilities can add up to something substantial. However, the total of all disabilities cannot exceed 100% plus allowances for a spouse, dependent children or dependent parents. In short, if you think you have any service-connected disabilities, it is prudent to get yourself into the VA system before you get Prostate Cancer so you can minimize negotiating the bureaucracy while trying to deal with the cancer.

D. File for Disability Compensation from the Veterans Administration as described in I.B. and I.C. (above). Even if little comes from your application, you will have your records organized, a VA File Number assigned and your service, particularly that in certain overseas areas, verified. All these could speed up a Prostate Cancer disability claim, should you be diagnosed at a later date. Having these things behind you can allow you to focus more on your treatment and less on covering your out-of-pocket expenses, which can be substantial. Doing this also provides an opportunity to establish a relationship with your local veteran service office that could be most beneficial if you should need assistance in the future.

2

My Story

Like many, if not most, men of my generation, I know little about medicine or biology and didn't worry much about my health---until getting hit with the cosmic two by four, that is. The blunt object that struck my head was a PSA score of 6.3 in December 2009, a couple of months after my 63rd birthday. I had never had a PSA test, digital rectal exam, or anything of the like and wasn't too keen on the idea. My family doctor informed me that, although the level was a good bit higher than the "normal" range of zero to 4, he had seen patients with PSAs of up to 15 who didn't have Prostate Cancer as PSAs aren't perfect indicators. He then gave me my first digital rectal examination (DRE)---which wasn't as bad as I feared---and found nothing unusual. He then suggested that I see a urologist and gave me a list---a short list because I live in a small town---of local urologists he considers competent. I arbitrarily selected one and made an appointment.

The first thing I had to learn was what PSA stands for. Prostate-specific antigen (PSA) is a protein produced only by the prostate gland. Normally, only a small amount of PSA escapes to circulate in a man's bloodstream. Prostate Cancer causes considerably more PSA to be found in the blood. The PSA Test is far from a perfect measure as many false positives are produced and some cancerous tumors are missed, but it is the best indicator available at present.

I didn't realize that urologists like to start with a urine test, and I failed to "study" for it before going to his office. After drinking a lot of water, I eventually passed that test. I also passed his DRE. Finding nothing obvious and having no baseline PSA to compare against, the urologist scheduled me for a biopsy. That was an adventure. I won't go into the prep work for the procedure except to say that sanitary work areas tend to result in fewer infections; I paid a good bit of attention on cleaning that area before leaving home for the biopsy.

Biopsies, at least where I live, are generally done as outpatient procedures in facilities often associated with urologists, though not necessarily in their offices. There are three general modes of collecting tissue samples for prostate cancer biopsies. The type most commonly performed in South Central Pennsylvania, where I live, is the transrectal ultrasound guided prostate biopsy. The urologist inserted both the ultrasound probe and sampling gun into the rectum while I was awake. A local anesthetic jelly was used to reduce the discomfort. Although not very painful, the procedure was quite uncomfortable. It seemed to take quite a long time for him to extract the 12 core samples from my prostate. Each core sample is quite small in diameter, that of the 18-gauge needle used to extract it, and less than an inch long, so site selection is important in picking locations that might sample cancerous tumors if they are present. My prostate had no lumps or other visible signs to guide him toward sites that were likely cancerous. The procedure seemed to take forever but probably only took 45 minutes.

Because the prostate is located adjacent to the colon but outside of it, the ultrasound is needed to present the urologist with a fairly clear picture of it. But to actually take the samples, the colon's wall must be punctured to extract each core. The side effects of this procedure were underplayed, in my opinion, as the bleeding in my urine and semen continued for several weeks as did the painful ejaculation. I was relieved, however, when the lab results, which I never saw, came back negative. He said that my prostate was a fair amount larger than average but showed no signs of problems. Getting that good news made the inconvenience seem worthwhile. Life then went on as usual. After all, high PSA readings are normal for many men and can be caused by several things besides prostate cancer.

That was April, 2010. The following December, I was shocked to hear that my annual PSA test showed a value of 8.8. Such a large change in just a year is cause for alarm. I asked my family physician to have a new test run, which he did. This time, the PSA was 10.2! He then requested that a Free PSA Test be run on that same sample to get a better idea of the likelihood that prostate cancer was causing the high readings. That test compares the portion of the PSA that circulates freely in the blood against the amount that is attached to protein molecules. That test was inconclusive in showing whether I had Prostate Cancer or not. The date was Thursday, December 23, two days before Christmas. I called the urologist and left a message. I got no reply. Not getting a reply the next day, Christmas Eve, was not unexpected but was a bit disconcerting. Only getting his answering service again on the Monday after Christmas didn't help things a bit, so I called again on Tuesday morning but got no response. By this time, I was getting frantic. I asked my family physician to intervene on my behalf. While waiting for the results of his intervention, I ran some errands, one of which took me near the urologist's office. So, I dropped in. It was locked up tight as if closed for vacation. When my family physician had no better success at reaching the urologist, I asked him to get me an appointment with another local urologist as soon as possible. I left a message with the first urologist's answering service stating that, if he wanted to keep me as a patient, he should call me by the close of business that day. He didn't. My family physician got me an appointment with another urologist for first thing the following Monday morning, the first workday after New Year's. The first urologist's office finally called me back on Wednesday the 29th to see if they should have him call me. I simply told her that it would not be necessary.

The second urologist was young and personable as was the first but was located in less impressive quarters. His practice is associated in some way with the local hospital, a reason why his fairly new office is rather institutional in appearance. Since I am one of those people who pays for his own health insurance complete with high deductibles and co-payments, lavish quarters were not desirable if they translated into higher rates. After looking over the PSA tests, the new urologist conducted the dreaded DRE and noted that my prostate felt to be larger than normal and a bit hard, possibly due to the recent biopsy. Due largely to the rapidly increasing PSA, he recommended a second biopsy. That was delayed to the 26th because my world-traveling wife had already scheduled us for a two-week trip to Morocco. That biopsy went better than the first one because it seemed to be over much more quickly and the side effects didn't last as long.

We left to escape the snow and cold on the evening of January 31 as we do part of each winter. While we were driving through Georgia the next day, the urologist called with the preliminary results. The pathologist at the local hospital had found a small amount of low-grade cancer in one of the 12 cores. So, I had prostate cancer! That was not the best news I ever received, not by a long shot. Being in Florida for a month before I could meet with either the urologist or my family doctor gave me time to think about things.

I started doing some research about the various treatment modalities that are available. The good news was that, because my cancer appeared to have been detected at a very early stage and hadn't likely spread beyond the prostate, I was a pretty good candidate for all of these treatment types, all of which would save my life if administered competently. The bad news was that most of the treatments had some pretty nasty side effects, with incontinence and impotency being two of the worst and most common. I started calling people who I knew who had been treated for prostate cancer. Most had chosen radical surgery or radiation therapy, the most common treatments, at least where I live. Though satisfied that their treatments had saved their lives, all of them stated that they were no long the people they were before the treatment. I decided to do more research.

After returning from Florida, I met with both doctors separately on successive days. Both recommended watchful waiting because the cancer was deemed as being in an early stage of development and that the side-effects were nasty in the best case and horrendous in the worst. I did not want to end up wearing a diaper for the rest of my life. More research was definitely needed and it appeared that I needed to not rush a decision. Time was a luxury of which I had a bit.

Eventually, I came across something that wasn't widely available but looked very promising, proton therapy. The more I read about it, the more curious I got. After discovering that Indiana University had a proton therapy center in Bloomington, where I attended grad school some years ago, I contacted them. The people with whom I talked were friendly and most helpful. Dr. Buchsbaum even took time out of his busy schedule to answer some of my questions. They mailed me a packet of information that was most informative. Included in the packet was a book, *You Can Beat Prostate Cancer And You Don't Need Surgery to Do It* by Robert J. Marckini. This book was written from the perspective of a patient who happened to be an analytical type as I am. His book and his methodology resonated with me. It also filled in some blank spaces in my own research. After reading his book, I contacted some men who had had proton therapy and found that they had had similar experiences to those of the people mentioned in the book. I was pretty well convinced that proton therapy offered me the best chance at a high quality of life after treatment of all the treatment modalities available. I could deal with having a formerly cancerous prostate still in my body after treatment was over. Some men with whom I spoke just had to have their prostates removed surgically because they felt they needed to have them out of their bodies. Proton therapy was definitely not for them. No one treatment is for everyone. Convinced that it was for me, I scheduled an interview at the Indiana University Health Proton Therapy Center in Bloomington on April 14, 2011.

Dr. Jeffrey Buchsbaum reviewed my medical reports and confirmed that I was a good candidate for proton therapy. He also informed me that I was a prime candidate for the other modalities as well. That was reassuring. Immediately before the interview, I was measured to make sure that I wasn't too fat for the machine. IU's system is unique due to its genesis and the design of its cyclotron (Proton therapy requires either a cyclotron or particle accelerator to extract protons from the nuclei of atoms). It can treat longer areas than can some other installations but cannot treat as deeply as some. The IU Physics Department had a cyclotron in Bloomington (IU's medical school is in Indianapolis) that they used for experiments for NASA. After the NASA contracts ran out, they repurposed the cyclotron for medical use at a fraction of the usual cost for building such an installation. IU got a proton therapy center on the cheap, $45M in this case, and I am a beneficiary of their good fortune. However, much remained to be done before my good fortune could be realized.

First off was finding a way to pay for this expensive treatment. All prostate cancer treatments are expensive but, not counting after-treatment costs, proton therapy is the most expensive of all due to the large capital investment required for an installation and the large number of treatments prescribed, often numbering 44. For most people, health insurance is required to pay for the bulk of the cost of the major treatments. Fortunately for me, Highmark Blue Cross/Blue Shield agreed to cover it. I have the regular retail fee-for-services policy that is available for anyone to buy. An advantage to this policy is that there are fewer restrictions limiting providers that I'm allowed to use than PPOs and, especially, HMOs generally have. I've read that Medicare has been covering proton therapy but may be under pressure to stop due to its high initial cost. That proton therapy patients don't usually require follow-up surgeries to correct problems in the urinary tract or prescriptions for drugs such as Viagra offsets the difference in initial cost a good bit. However, health insurance doesn't cover travel and living expenses, which can be significant.

A chance reading of a letter to the editor led to finding a way to cover out-of-pocket expenses associated with my treatment. While driving to Florida just hours before learning that I had prostate cancer, my wife read the then current issue of a diabetes magazine I had received as a gift from a friend after being diagnosed with Type II Diabetes. A short letter to the editor pointed out that veterans who served in Vietnam and had Type II Diabetes were eligible for disabilities from the Veterans Administration (VA) because that was one of the diseases determined to have been the result of exposure to Agent Orange. After arriving in Florida, I visited the VA web site and found a list of diseases associated with Agent Orange. The list included both Type II Diabetes and Prostate Cancer. Boy! I have two Agent Orange-related diseases and didn't think I had been exposed to it. The F-102 fighter jets I had worked on at Bien Hoa Air Base were not capable of spraying defoliants, and I was never out in the bush. So, I thought I was safe and that the VA's willingness to provide me with a disability for these diseases was just a happy coincidence. I would learn more about that later.

The VA web site, www.va.gov, has a link to VONAPP (Veterans On-Line Application), a site where veterans' disability claims can be filed. After reading that benefits begin on the date the application is filed, not the date the disease was diagnosed, I filed the form, even though I didn't have all the necessary information at hand. Even the VA admits that they take many months to evaluate a claim to determine eligibility but make payments retroactive to the date the claim was filed. So, it behooved me to get the application in as soon as possible, even though it was incomplete. Recalling that the physician who gave me my discharge physical in 1969 said that the hearing in my right ear was diminished and knowing that I had spent most of my time in the Air Force working on the flightline in close proximity to jets with their engines running, I included hearing loss and the tinnitus (ringing in my ears) that appeared later in the list of health problems related to my Air Force service. Other than my DD-214, and the Prostate Cancer lab report, I didn't have much in the way of documentation with me to submit with the initial application. I wouldn't be home for a month, so it was better to get the process started than to hold off until everything was available.

Like most of my peers, I was just a kid of 19 when I went into the service and didn't know much about anything, particularly about the need to keep important papers. Not knowing they would be needed in the future, I didn't keep copies of my orders or much else. So, I requested a copy of my file from the Air Force Records Center. They arrived some weeks later but, not surprisingly, were not complete. The VA requires three major items to determine Agent Orange eligibility: 1) documentation that one served on the ground in Vietnam between January 9, 1962 and May 7, 1975 for however short a time period, 2) that one was discharged for other than dishonorable conditions, and 3) medical diagnosis of an Agent Orange-related disease. My DD-214 indicated that I had an honorable discharge, so it satisfied the second criteria. The box for decorations and medals listed VSM (Vietnam Service Medal), but it is my understanding that some people stationed in Thailand also received the VSM. It listed my dates of service as being from May 10, 1966 to December 26, 1969, well within the date range specified by criteria one. So, the DD-214 was incomplete in satisfying the first criteria. I already had the pathologist's interim report on my biopsy which should have satisfied the third criteria for Prostate Cancer. A little later, I received the final report and a second opinion on the biopsy from Johns Hopkins, both of which confirmed the preliminary diagnosis. I already had a letter from my family physician from a year earlier in which he informed me that I was diagnosed as having Type II Diabetes, another Agent Orange-related disease, and prescribed Metformin to treat it. It appeared that all I was lacking was a copy of the orders that sent me to Bien Hoa Air Base. My Air Force file included a copy of the orders on which sent me to Don Muang Air Base, Thailand, but not one for Vietnam. This was a significant gap in my documentation.

After wracking my brain quite awhile, I recalled that a Tech Sergeant from my shop traveled with me to Bien Hoa. Eventually, I figured out how to spell his last name. I remembered his first name so that wasn't a problem. Some research using www.zabasearch.com found a person with that name, about 12 years older than me living in Port St. Lucie, Florida. I called the number and asked the retired Master Sergeant who answered the phone if he had worked in the MG-10 shop at Clark AFB. When he answered yes, I knew I had found the right person. He didn't remember me but clearly recalled going to Bien Hoa at the time I recalled going there. He even mentioned some special duties he performed while assigned there. Being career military, he knew to keep copies of his orders and had his files close by. He put down the phone to look through the files but returned quickly with a paper. He read off, "Benjey, Thomas R. AF1686..." and I knew he had it. He scanned the sheet and emailed it to me. A short time later, I had the evidence I needed to satisfy the first criteria!

When I said I was skeptical about being exposed to Agent Orange, he was surprised that I hadn't noticed the C-123s taxiing by our row of revetments with defoliant dripping from their spray bars. I clearly recall the C-123s but didn't realize they had been spraying Agent Orange. The sergeant informed me that, on an open area on the ramp next to the U-2 hangar, airmen pumped Agent Orange into tanks in the C-123s from 55-gallon drums. I thought the C-123s were called Ranch Hands, so I was surprised to find out they were actually called Providers. Then I learned that the Agent Orange defoliation effort was called Operation Ranch Hand and Bien Hoa Air Base was a major hub for the spraying. The Vietnamese government placed Bien Hoa, Da Nang and Phu Cat air bases on a list for future cleanup of the residual Agent Orange in those sites. I was not at Da Nang during the war, but many others from my outfit were.

After mailing the supporting documentation for eligibility to the VA Regional Office, I was ready to learn more about the benefits of a VA Disability. Prostate Cancer disabilities appear to be treated differently than other types, possibly because the disease can be treated successfully by either killing the cancer cells or removing the prostate from the body. However, serious side effects often remain. The VA assigns a disability of 100% beginning on the later of two dates: the date of application or the date of diagnosis of Prostate Cancer. The veteran then receives monthly disability payments, depending on his marital status and number of dependent children or parents. These payments continue until six months after treatment of his cancer is complete. (It is unclear how patients who choose watchful waiting are handled.) The veteran is re-examined at this time to determine the continuing disability, if any, from residual effects of the Prostate Cancer or as a result of the treatment. Residual effects can range from frequent urination, waking up at night to urinate, to incontinence and impotence.

After providing the VA Regional Office all the documentation I had, they scheduled me for an examination at Lebanon Veterans Hospital in Lebanon, Pennsylvania. Actually, they gave me five appointments on one day with the first one being at 8:45 a.m. at a lab. I assumed that they would be taking blood for a PSA Test and a Hemoglobin A 1 c Test to help confirm that I had Prostate Cancer and Type II Diabetes, respectively. The 9:30 appointment was at C&P AUD, which I interpreted to be the Compensation and Pension audio lab to assess my hearing and tinnitus. The 10:45 appointment was with the C&P CLERK whom, I assumed, would take any additional paperwork I might have. At 11:00 a.m., I was scheduled to meet with C&P CARLSON. Perhaps a Dr. Carlson would examine me for the various conditions I have. The last appointment was at 1:20 p.m. in the X-RAY Clinic. I had no idea what they planned to do then.

The VA examination turned out to be less stressful than it might have been. Waiting times were relatively short and the people there were generally cordial if a bit officious. The lab technician took blood as expected and also a urine sample. It would have been nice if they would have warned me about that so I could have studied for the urine test. The technician said they were going to run the standard battery of tests, whatever that comprises. The woman in the audio lab tested my hearing extensively and said that, although my record shows some damage was done while I was in the Air Force, it is still pretty good. As far as the tinnitus goes, she found a scrap of paper in my file from 1968 when I apparently complained about the ringing in my ears at that time. She thought I'd probably get a small disability for that. Somewhere I read that would probably be 10%. It was my understanding that disabilities had to total at least 10% before the VA would compensate for them.

The C&P CLERK appointment amounted to a clerk filling in some missing data on the forms and didn't take long. Mr. Carlson informed me that he was conducting an examination for legal rather than medical purposes. He was interested more about my general health than the conditions about which I was complaining. He even took my blood pressure three times, something he said was a requirement. The last examination was a chest x-ray, which Mr. Carlson instructed me to get immediately so that he would have everything necessary to file a report on me before he left for vacation that afternoon. He also suggested that I sign a Release of Information form at the ROI Office for the x-rays so that copies would be sent to my primary care physician and informed me that, if I stopped at the Travel Office, the VA would reimburse me for my mileage to and from the hospital that day. The x-rays didn't take long, nor did the other two stops. I was on my way an hour before the X-RAY Clinic was scheduled. Not a bad experience for the first time at a VA hospital, all things considered. Mr. Carlson was hesitant to make predictions, particularly about the future, but figured it would be some months before the VA made a decision. Shortly after starting treatment, I contacted the VA again, two weeks after their examination, but found out nothing except that I should have the treating physician fax them his notes on diagnosis and treatment.

Not thinking it wise to delay treatment while waiting for a decision from the VA, I proceeded with scheduling proton therapy in Indiana. Treatment for Prostate Cancer often involves several preliminary procedures. In my case, that included a CT scan and a bone scan at my local hospital to make sure the cancer had not spread outside the prostate. A colonoscopy determined that I didn't have polyps or rectal cancer. In Indiana, a gold seed was inserted in my prostate to be used in aiming the radiation at my prostate more precisely. A cast was made of my midsection from which a plastic pod was made to hold me in the same position during each treatment. Another CT scan, this time in the pod and with the gold seed present, and an MRI were made for the physicians and technicians to assist in developing my treatment plan. So, I was a busy guy for over a month getting ready for the treatment. On June 22, I had my V-Sim or dress rehearsal and actual treatments began on June 23.

As of this writing, I have completed the 44- treatment regime---with no significant side effects. During the treatments, I felt nothing from the radiation. Fortunately, the machine clicks as it is doing its thing so I know when it starts and stops. So far, so good. Now to get the VA to chip in to help cover my mounting medical and travel costs. It's seven months since I first applied, so I call them every other week to check on the status. Early on, they identified additional documentation they desired. Persistence is the watchword when dealing with government agencies. On July 28, the VA informed me that they had not received the documents related to my treatment Indiana University Health Proton Therapy Center faxed to them on July 1. Veterans' support web sites recommend sending documents to the VA via certified mail return receipt requested. So, I resent the missing documentation via certified mail return receipt requested. On August 19, the Rating Board made a decision on my claim and on September 8, the VA decision letter arrived stating that a lump-sum check would be sent in 15 days and monthly checks the beginning of each month after that. The VA took seven months to process my claim less, I'm told, than many others take.

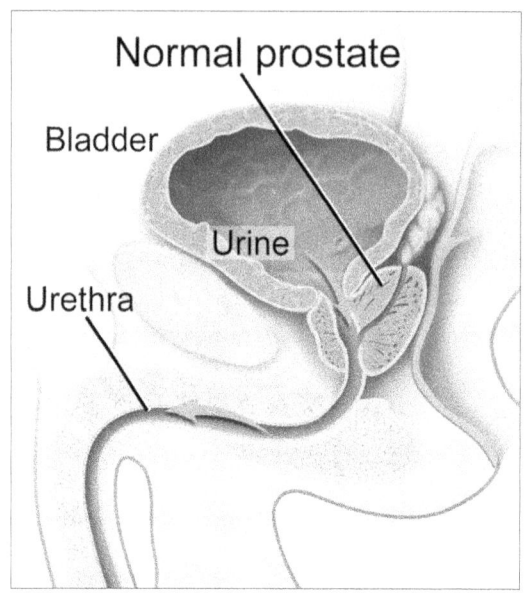

It not uncommon for men with prostate cancer to have enlarged prostate glands as well.

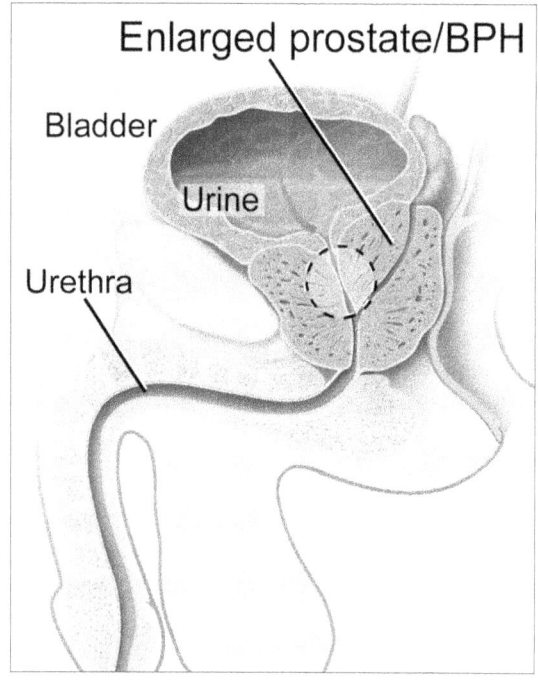

Drawings Courtesy National Cancer Institute.

3

VA Disabilities

Since 1930, the Veterans Administration has had the responsibility of caring for U. S. military veterans injured in the service of their country. However, the level and quality of care has varied. For years, Vietnam veterans reported numerous illnesses after returning home from the "conflict," but their claims were denied by the Veterans Administration. Over time, the VA has been forced to reassess its position. A 2008 study conducted by physicians at the University of California Davis Cancer Center showed that Vietnam veterans who were exposed to Agent Orange have greatly increased risks of getting Prostate Cancer and even greater risks of getting the most aggressive form of the disease than those who were not exposed. A 2009 study conducted on 1,663 veterans at five different VA medical centers who had previously undergone surgical removal of their prostates found that the 206 known to have been exposed to Agent Orange had an almost 50 percent increased risk of their cancer recurring than the others and the cancer that returned was much more aggressive.

I. Agent Orange Diseases

Approximately 3,000,000 American service people, primarily men, served in Vietnam during the Vietnam War. Agent Orange was used to defoliate forests and other potential battlegrounds from 1962 to 1975, with the greatest concentration of spraying occurring between 1967 and 1969, peak years in troop deployment. About 1.5 million service people served in Vietnam during this peak spraying period. The VA is now reimbursing veterans for disabilities believed to be the result of exposure to Agent Orange, and Prostate Cancer is one of the diseases covered by this disability program. In order to qualify for an Agent Orange disability, one must demonstrate:

1. That he served on the ground in Vietnam between January 9, 1962 and May 7, 1975, and

2. That he has been diagnosed with Prostate Cancer.

Additionally, "Brown Water Veterans" who served on inland waterways on patrol and swift boats and "Blue Water Veterans" who went ashore when their ships docked in Vietnam or who served aboard ships that operated on the inland waterways are also deemed eligible. Veterans who served in Korea between April 1, 1968 and August 31, 1971 in or near the demilitarized zone are believed to have been exposed, too; they are also eligible for a disability if they have Prostate Cancer.

In addition to Prostate Cancer, a veteran may have other illnesses, including Agent Orange diseases. The VA also deems Agent Orange veterans as qualified for disabilities if they have any of these diseases:

- **Acute and Subacute Peripheral Neuropathy**
  A nervous system condition that causes numbness, tingling, and motor weakness. Under VA's rating regulations, it must be at least 10% disabling within 1 year of exposure to herbicides and resolve within 2 years after the date it began.
- **AL Amyloidosis**
  A rare disease caused when an abnormal protein, amyloid, enters tissues or organs.
- **Chloracne (or Similar Acneform Disease)**
  A skin condition that occurs soon after exposure to chemicals and looks like common forms of acne seen in teenagers. Under VA's rating regulations, chloracne (or other acneform disease similar to chloracne) must be at least 10% disabling within 1 year of exposure to herbicides.
- **Chronic B-cell Leukemias**
  A type of cancer which affects white blood cells. VA's regulation recognizing all chronic B-cell leukemias as related to exposure to herbicides took effect on October 30, 2010.

- **Diabetes Mellitus (Type 2)**
  A disease characterized by high blood sugar levels resulting from the body's inability to respond properly to the hormone insulin.
- **Hodgkin's Disease**
  A malignant lymphoma (cancer) characterized by progressive enlargement of the lymph nodes, liver, and spleen, and by progressive anemia.
- **Ischemic Heart Disease**
  A disease characterized by a reduced supply of blood to the heart, that leads to chest pain. VA's regulation recognizing ischemic heart disease as related to exposure to herbicides took effect on October 30, 2010.
- **Multiple Myeloma**
  A cancer of plasma cells, a type of white blood cell in bone marrow.
- **Non-Hodgkin's Lymphoma**
  A group of cancers that affect the lymph glands and other lymphatic tissue.
- **Parkinson's Disease**
  A progressive disorder of the nervous system that affects muscle movement. VA's regulation recognizing Parkinson's disease as related to exposure to herbicides took effect on October 30, 2010.
- **Porphyria Cutanea Tarda**
  A disorder characterized by liver dysfunction and by thinning and blistering of the skin in sun-exposed areas. Under VA's rating regulations, it must be at least 10% disabling within 1 year of exposure to herbicides.
- **Prostate Cancer**
  Cancer of the prostate; one of the most common cancers among men.
- **Respiratory Cancers**
  Cancers of the lung, larynx, trachea, and bronchus.

- **Soft Tissue Sarcoma (other than Osteosarcoma, Chondrosarcoma, Kaposi's sarcoma, or Mesothelioma)**
A group of different types of cancers in body tissues such as muscle, fat, blood and lymph vessels, and connective tissues.

II. Disability Payments

After examining veterans who apply for a disability, the VA assigns them a percentage from zero to 100, depending on what they observe in the examination and the documentation the veteran provides. Partial disabilities may be summed together, but the total cannot exceed 100%. Depending on whether he is single or married or has dependent children or parents, the veteran receives a monthly disability payment from the tables that follow:

(No Dependents)

Percentage	Rate
10%	$123
20%	$243

Without Children

Dependent Status	30%	40%	50%	60%
Veteran Alone	$376	$541	$770	$974
Veteran with Spouse Only	$421	$601	$845	$1064
Veteran with Spouse & One Parent	$457	$649	$905	$1136
Veteran with Spouse and Two Parents	$493	$697	$965	$1208
Veteran with One Parent	$412	$589	$830	$1046
Veteran with Two Parents	$448	$637	$890	$1118
Additional for A/A spouse (see footnote b)	$40	$54	$68	$81

Without Children

Dependent Status	70%	80%	90%	100%
Veteran Alone	$1,228	$1,427	$1,604	$2,673
Veteran with Spouse Only	$1,333	$1,547	$1,739	$2,823
Veteran with Spouse & One Parent	$1,417	$1,643	$1,847	$2,943
Veteran with Spouse and Two Parents	$1,501	$1,739	$1,955	$3,063
Veteran with One Parent	$1,312	$1,523	$1,712	$2,793
Veteran with Two Parents	$1,396	$1,619	$1,820	$2,913
Additional for A/A spouse (see footnote b)	$95	$108	$122	$136

With Children

Dependent Status	30%	40%	50%	60%
Veteran with Spouse & Child	$453	$644	$899	$1129
Veteran with Child Only	$406	$581	$820	$1034
Veteran with Spouse, One Parent and Child	$489	$692	$959	$1201
Veteran with Spouse, Two Parents and Child	$525	$740	$1019	$1,273
Veteran with One Parent and Child	$442	$629	$880	$1106
Veteran with Two Parents and Child	$478	$677	$940	$1178
Add for Each Additional Child Under Age 18	$22	$30	$37	$45
Each Additional Schoolchild Over Age 18 (see footnote a)	$72	$96	$120	$144
Additional for A/A spouse (see footnote b)	$40	$54	$68	$81

With Children

Dependent Status	70%	80%	90%	100%
Veteran with Spouse & Child	$1,409	$1,634	$1,837	$2,932
Veteran with Child Only	$1,298	$1,507	$1,694	$2,774
Veteran with Spouse, One Parent and Child	$1,493	$1,730	$1,945	$3,052
Veteran with Spouse, Two Parents and Child	$1,577	$1,826	$2,053	$3,172
Veteran with One Parent and Child	$1,382	$1,603	$1,802	$2,894
Veteran with Two Parents and Child	$1,466	$1,699	$1,910	$3,014

Add for Each Additional Child Under Age 18	$52	$60	$67	$75
Each Additional Schoolchild Over Age 18 (footnote a)	$168	$192	$216	$240
Additional for A/A spouse (see footnote b)	$95	$108	$122	$136

FOOTNOTES:

a. For each school child are shown separately. They are not included with any other compensation rates. All other entries on this chart reflecting a rate for children show the rate payable for children under 18 or helpless. To find the amount payable to a 70% disabled veteran with a spouse and four children, one of whom is over 18 and attending school, take the 70% rate for a veteran with a spouse and 3 children, $1,513, and add the rate for one school child, $168. The total amount payable is $1,681.

b. The veteran has a spouse who is determined to require A/A, add the figure shown as "additional for A/A spouse" to the amount shown for the proper dependency code. For example, veteran has A/A spouse and 2 minor children and is 70% disabled. Add $95, additional for A/A spouse, to the rate for a 70% veteran with dependency code 12, $1,461. The total amount payable is $ 1,556.

It is the author's understanding that retired military personnel are eligible for disability payments and the offset against retired pay will be phased out by 2014. Apparently Agent-Orange disabilities are not subject to this phase-out period. It is also his understanding that VA disability payments are non-taxable income.

A July 2011 news report indicated that the VA now pays for caregiver support for veterans disabled so badly that they cannot attend to daily life functions on their own. Most vets with prostate cancer will catch it early enough and get competent treatment, making having a caregiver unnecessary. However, for those cases in which the cancer progresses to the point that assistance with basic functions is required, the VA now provides financial support for caregivers, including family members. Qualifying for such support is not easy and requires completion of the Comprehensive Assistance for Family Caregivers course. Caregiver support can be applied for on-line at www.va.gov/healtheligibility/caregiver/Q4NoNotEnrolled.asp.

4
Treatment Modalities for Prostate Cancer

When Prostate Cancer is detected early in its development, the broadest range of treatment modalities is available to the patient. If the cancer spreads, the options narrow significantly. Fortunately, these days Prostate Cancer tends to be found fairly early in most patients, so all of these modalities are open to a great number of patients. Personal factors can limit the treatments an individual might consider. Some men absolutely must have their prostates removed for psychological reasons. Merely killing the cancerous cells is not acceptable. For them, some type of surgery or ablation is the only acceptable approach. Working men who need their income to continue uninterrupted and cannot afford to be away from their jobs for more than a few days must choose treatments within easy commuting distance or that require a minimum of time off work. Thus, proton therapy is not currently a choice for the majority of working men because it is available only at a few locations. Radiation or IMRT require about the same number of treatments as proton therapy (short daily sessions for about 9 weeks that can be done before or after work) but are offered in even small towns, thus making them viable options. Urologists tend to specialize in a specific treatment approach and group practices usually offer just a few, often surgery and radiation. Men who have developed confidence in their urologist may feel they will get better care from him or her and choose the modality in which he or she specializes.

Not all insurance companies cover all modalities. And ablation is not covered by most insurers as yet. Due to the costly nature of these treatments, insurance coverage is essential. My advice would be to ignore the cost at first and determine which treatment would give you the best realistic chance of the outcome you want. Then, ask the provider to assist with getting your insurer to cover it. Only accept your second choice after exhausting all options for getting you first choice. It's your life and you have to live with the results and side effects; the younger you are, the longer you will have to live with them.

The choice you make may not affect only you. If you are married, it also affects your wife. So, she must be involved in the decision-making process and should be informed. Even better, she should read Robert Marckini's book. Chapter 6 treats the various options so well that I refer you to his book and only summarize them here.

I. Watchful Waiting

No treatment is made but periodic PSA Tests and less frequent biopsies are made to determine if and when treatment is advised.

<u>Advantages</u>

Least intrusive and least expensive approach. Slow-growing nature of many prostate cancers may not ever require treatment in elderly patients. Puts off trauma of treatment and potentially nasty side effects. Superior modalities may be developed during waiting period.

<u>Disadvantages</u>

Doesn't eliminate cancer from the body. May be difficult psychologically for some men. The cancer may spread more quickly than expected. Not a long-term solution for the non-elderly.

II. Surgery (Radical Prostatectomy)

The entire prostate gland is cut out of the body by the surgeon either with a knife or with the assistance of a robot. The most difficult part seems to be sparing the nerves that run alongside the prostate and control erectile function. Saving them is critical in reducing the erectile dysfunction that accompanies the removal of the prostate. The success of the surgery in removing the cancer and in minimizing unwanted side effects is, in significant part, due to the skill of the surgeon. Picking a skillful surgeon is a critically important decision if you select surgery for your treatment.

Advantages

A skilled surgeon can remove the cancer and save your life. If the cancer was confined to the prostate, it is gone for good. A highly skilled surgeon can save some of the nerves and greatly reduce the side effects of incontinence and impotence.

Disadvantages

Significant effort may be required to learn to control sphincter to regain continence after surgery. Overcoming impotence may require Viagra-like medications and/or other procedures, equipment or medicines. Worst case is wearing diapers the rest of your life for incontinence and being impotent.

III. External Beam Radiation

Radiation has been used to kill cancer for over 70 years. The type of radiation most commonly employed is photon radiation (x-rays) aimed from outside the body at the tumor inside the body. Higher dose rates have higher cure rates. Newer Intensity Modulated Radiation Therapy (IMRT) directs higher intensity beams at the thicker part of the tumor and lower intensity beams at thinner parts to reduce radiation exposure to surrounding healthy tissue.

Advantages

No hospital stay required. Will not need local anesthesia or be put to sleep. May have fewer urination problems than with surgery. Can often be done locally while continuing to work at your job as usual.

Disadvantages

Doesn't eliminate cancer from the body. May be difficult psychologically for some men. Sometimes necessary to have hormone treatment before radiation treatment to reduce testosterone that prostate cancer feeds on, thus eliminating libido. Libido may be slow in returning after treatment. Radiation treatment has similar erectile dysfunction issues as with surgery, but they tend to appear 3 to 5 years after treatment. One-third of men treated with radiation see their PSAs rise within 5 years of treatment and require further treatment if they are young and healthy enough.

IV. Brachytherapy

Urologist implants radioactive seeds or tiny catheters into the prostate or surrounding area. Seeds give off radiation to kill the cancer and remain in the body after giving off all the radiation. Catheters receive about 3 charges of radiation over a 24-hr period before they are removed.

<u>Advantages</u>

Success rates similar to conventional radiation. No overnight stay in hospital for seeds treatment. Much less invasive than surgery. Less radiation damage to surrounding organ and tissue than with external beam radiation.

<u>Disadvantages</u>

Doesn't eliminate cancer from the body. May be difficult psychologically for some men. Risk of impotence and incontinence similar to those with surgery. Seeds sometimes come loose and travel to other parts of the body. Some men have had seeds reach their lungs and others have had problems with seeds settling into their hip joints. I'm told seeds are now being strung together to prevent migration.

V. Cryotherapy

Cryotherapy involves killing the cancer tumor by freezing it. It is less invasive than most other treatments and often requires no overnight hospital stay. It is effective in the early stages of prostate cancer with low risk for tumor extension.

<u>Advantages</u>

Less intrusive than surgery with good cure rates and can be used if cancer recurs after another treatment. Overnight hospital stay often not required.

<u>Disadvantages</u>
Risk of recurrence. Little long-term data is available because Cryotherapy is a relatively new treatment.

VI. Proton Therapy

Proton therapy involves separating protons from the nuclei of atoms and aiming them at the prostate gland. Because protons operate according to the Bragg Peak, they can be more accurately aimed at tumors and cause less damage to healthy tissue. Like other radiations, proton therapy requires short treatments for eight or nine weeks.

<u>Advantages</u>
Less intrusive than some other methods with fewer side effects during and after treatment. Less healthy tissue destroyed than with other radiation therapies. Offers otherwise healthy men a good shot at a full life after treatment.

<u>Disadvantages</u>
Expensive because proton therapy requires a cyclotron or particle accelerator. Few installations currently in place and few more planned due to cost. Requires that patient be within daily commuting distance for treatment. Some insurance companies don't cover it.

There is now hope for veterans who get their healthcare through the VA to receive proton therapy for their Prostate Cancer. I recently learned that the Indianapolis and Philadelphia VA offices on occasion send patients to proton therapy centers not in their system as the VA has no proton therapy centers. If you think proton therapy is the right treatment for you, press the VA, if necessary, to have you treated with proton therapy at one of the growing number of centers around the country.

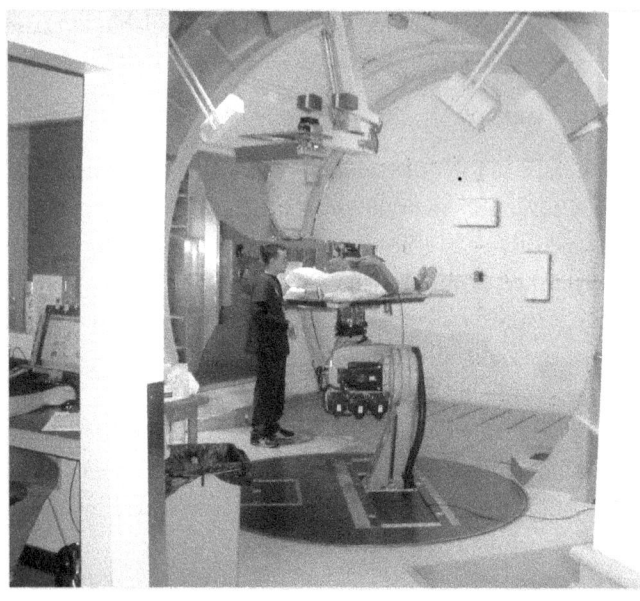

Author being positioned for proton therapy treatment. Photo © Ann Benjey.

5

Cost

One of the things that the various treatment modalities have in common is that they're costly—very costly and rising. And we're not talking about thousands of dollars; we're talking about tens or hundreds of thousands. A reason for the large and escalating prices is the cost of the equipment now being used in treating Prostate Cancer patients. For example, removing diseased prostrates by surgery is commonly done these days with the assistance of robots, even at small-town hospitals such as the one in my home town. This equipment costs well over a million dollars to acquire and more than $100,000 a year for maintenance. I'm told that the cost of an external beam radiation system (IMRT) is in the same ballpark. Proton beam radiation systems generally cost in the hundreds of millions of dollars. Indiana University was able to build its system for a mere $45,000,000 because they already had a cyclotron that was available for repurposing for medical use. Equipment costs as well as labor costs associated with their use must be recouped from patients or their insurance companies.

Determining what a treatment will cost is a black art. Each provider has its usual and customary charge for each procedure it performs. Think of this as the list price or full retail or the price a wealthy person without insurance would pay. (Prostate cancer procedures are so expensive that a poor person without insurance would not likely be able to pay for it.) Providers negotiate discounted rates with insurance companies and Medicare. So, the insurer generally pays far less than list price for the procedure. However, insurance doesn't usually cover the entire amount that was negotiated; some of that is left to the insured. The insured is levied for co-pays and deductibles which vary from policy to policy, group to group, and employer to employer. In my case, I had a fairly high deductible policy. My total consisted of a $1,500 deductible and a 20% co-pay to a maximum of $6,000 or $7,500 per policy year. Most treatments are so expensive that they will probably max out your deductible and co-pay for the year. So, I don't think there is much difference in patient cost for the various treatment modalities, provided they are covered by insurance.

The per policy year stipulation is important because the counter is reset the first day of each policy year. My policy year began on June 1, three weeks before my treatment started. That means that any costs incurred prior to June 1 counted toward the previous year's total, not the total for my out-of-pocket expenses for the year of the treatment. The policy year is important because I was diagnosed at the beginning of the final third of my policy year, which means that the procedures leading up to the Prostrate Cancer treatment---biopsy, bonescan, CT scan, consultation and colonoscopy---all occurred in that plan year, not the plan year of the treatment. These were not inexpensive, so my total out-of-pocket expense for the cancer far exceeded the annual maximum. I don't regret it because I wanted to move forward and didn't want to push things back a few months. If you think you have plenty of time to do something about your cancer, you can schedule the preliminaries and the treatment so they all fall in the same policy year and save yourself some money.

My recommendation is to pick the treatment you are most comfortable with and not worry too much about the cost. The provider will probably negotiate with your insurance company for you to determine if they will cover your treatment. The insurer will also tell the provider what your out-of-pocket costs will be. If your treatment requires travel, keep track of all those costs, too, because your medical costs could easily exceed the 7.5% of Adjusted Gross Income (AGI) threshold and be deductible on that year's income tax. Note that this threshold increases to 10% on January 1, 2013 as a provision of the 2010 healthcare bill commonly called Obamacare. If you should be diagnosed in 2012, it may be to your financial detriment to put off your treatment. However, if you are 65 or over, this threshold increase is to be delayed until January 1, 2017 and will not be a factor for consideration until 2016.

It is my understanding that VA Disability payments are not taxable income and, as such, aren't included when computing your AGI. If it were included in the AGI, the threshold for deductibility, in dollar terms, would be raised. Fortunately, that doesn't appear to be the case. However, your disability money can be used to help offset your out-of-pocket expenses, which can be quite large, and make the more expensive treatments and those that require travel affordable. If you don't have insurance, there are still some options open. Many providers treat a few patients for free. Don't be shy in asking providers for financial assistance if you don't have insurance. Also, as a veteran, treatment may be available to you at a VA hospital at no, or little, cost to you. However, be very careful when being treated for prostate cancer by the VA. Beginning in 2002, the Philadelphia VA Hospital botched the implanting of radioactive seeds in 92 prostate cancer patients with horrendous results in some cases. No amount of restitution can make you whole again, so it is incumbent on you to be on top of everything the VA does or proposes to do to you.

6
Conclusions

Being diagnosed with Prostate Cancer need not be a death sentence If found in an early stage—and it can easily be if you have annual PSA tests—you can not only live but have a full life after treatment. If the cancer is more progressed, your life can be saved but you may have to live with undesirable side effects. So, keep on top of it. Chances are, if you're reading this book, you're old enough to have a PSA test done. If you haven't done so already, get tested today.

If you are a veteran, particularly one who served in Vietnam, the Veterans Administration has programs that can help you. Just follow the instructions in this book and be sure to send your documentation to the VA via certified mail return receipt requested. That way you can show the VA that the documents you sent were actually delivered to them. Some veterans have had Agent-Orange related claims denied because their prostate cancer did not appear within one year of discharge from the service. This misapplication of the law has apparently been the result of poor training or an attempt to quickly reduce the backlog of claims to be processed. Should this happen to your claim, it will be necessary for you to appeal the decision. Dealing with the VA can require much persistence. Take care.

www.ingramcontent.com/pod-product-compliance
Lightning Source LLC
Chambersburg PA
CBHW070037040426
42333CB00040B/1702